CANDIDA DIET

FOR NOVICES

Enriched Recipes, Foods, Meal Plan & Procedures That Focuses On Optimal Wellness, Transforming Health, Stress Reduction, Good Sleeping Habits And More

DR. MATEO GABRIEL

DISCLAIMER

The information in this book is only meant to be used for general reading. In any way, the author and publisher do not promise or represent that the information in this work is full, correct, reliable, appropriate, or available. This includes any warranties that are expressed or implied. Because of this, you should only rely on this material at your own risk.

This book is not meant to replace professional help. If you have any questions about a subject, you should always get help from a qualified expert. The author and distributor of this book are not responsible for how the information in it is used or abused.

The author's thoughts and feelings are shown in this book. They do not necessarily represent the official policy or stance of any other person, group, employer, or business.

Any third-party material that you can get to through this book is not endorsed or backed by the author or publisher.

The information in this book is correct at the time it was published, after all possible checks. However, the author and distributor are not responsible for any loss, damage, or inconvenience that may be caused by mistakes or omissions.

TABLE OF CONTENTS

CHAPTER ONE

INTRODUCTION TO CANDIDA DIET

A naturally occurring microbe called candida is found in the mouth, throat, and stomach among other areas of the human body. Although modest levels of Candida are usually innocuous, an overabundance of this yeast can cause a condition called Candidiasis, which can cause a variety of health problems. For those looking to keep up a healthy and balanced lifestyle, it is essential to comprehend the dynamics of Candida and yeast overgrowth.

YEAST OVERGROWTH AND CANDIDA OVERVIEW

When the body's microbiome is out of balance, yeast can multiply unchecked, leading to Candida overgrowth. A weak immune system, hormone fluctuations, the use of antibiotics, and a diet heavy in processed carbohydrates are some of the factors that might upset the delicate microbial balance. Candida overgrowth can cause recurrent infections, tiredness, gastrointestinal problems, and skin concerns.

Acknowledging the complex interplay between Candida overgrowth and the body's general health is crucial to treating the condition holistically. When present in the right quantities, candida is essential for digestion and the absorption of nutrients. However, too much Candida can damage the lining of the stomach, making it difficult for the body to absorb vital nutrients and fostering an inflammatory environment.

DIET IS CRUCIAL FOR MANAGING CANDIDA

Food is a key factor in controlling Candida overgrowth since some meals either encourage or impede the growth of this yeast. Removing or reducing sugar, refined carbs, and processed items from the diet is essential to starving Candida of its favorite fuel source. Candida primarily uses sugar as an energy source, so cutting back on sugar consumption can help starve the yeast and prevent it from growing as much.

Additionally, adding foods high in anti-inflammatory and antifungal properties to the diet will help the body's defenses against Candida overgrowth. Foods high in probiotics, like yogurt and fermented veggies, help to rebuild a healthy gut microbiota by bringing in good bacteria that can outcompete and inhibit the growth of Candida.

CHAPTER TWO
RECOGNIZING CANDIDA
DESCRIBE CANDIDA

The human body naturally contains a kind of yeast called candida, which is mostly found in the skin, mucous membranes, and digestive tract. The most prevalent species of this yeast is Candida albicans, which normally gets along well with other microorganisms in the body without posing any problems. But when the microbiological equilibrium is thrown off, Candida can overgrow and cause a host of health issues.

REASONS FOR CANDIDA OVERGROWTH AND RISK FACTORS

In addition to a compromised immune system, several other factors can also lead to Candida overgrowth. Diseases including diabetes, autoimmune illnesses, and HIV/AIDS might make it more difficult for the body to properly control yeast levels. Moreover, a common risk factor for Candida overgrowth is the use of broad-spectrum antibiotics, which have the potential to upset the body's bacterial balance. Additional contributing factors include a diet high in refined sugars and carbs, which create a perfect habitat for yeast development, and hormonal changes, such as those that occur during pregnancy or while taking oral contraceptives.

SYMPTOMS OF CANDIDA OVERGROWTH

It can be difficult to detect Candida overgrowth because its symptoms can appear in a variety of ways. Recurrent yeast infections, chronic weariness, gastrointestinal problems including gas and bloating, and skin disorders like rashes and itching are typical symptoms. An overgrowth of Candida can also cause mood swings, attention problems, and sugar cravings in its sufferers. Since these symptoms are frequently nonspecific and can coexist with those of other medical disorders, medical professionals must perform a comprehensive assessment to identify the underlying cause.

DIAGNOSING CANDIDA

Because the symptoms of Candida overgrowth are ambiguous, making a diagnosis can be challenging. To make a diagnosis, medical practitioners may use a mix of laboratory testing, physical examination, and medical history. To determine if Candida is present and how much of an overgrowth there is, testing for the presence of the infection can be performed on blood, stool, or affected region cultures. To obtain an accurate diagnosis, medical professionals must rule out other possible explanations of the symptoms, such as autoimmune illnesses or bacterial infections. To properly assess and treat a patient, a thorough grasp of the patient's medical history and symptoms must be obtained, which means that patient and healthcare provider collaboration is critical throughout the diagnostic process.

CHAPTER THREE

BASICS OF THE CANDIDA DIET

DIET'S FUNCTION IN CANDIDA CONTROL

The overpopulation of the fungus Candida in the body causes a condition known as Candida overgrowth, which is managed and controlled mostly by following a diet high in Candida. The basic idea of the Candida diet is to limit the consumption of items that encourage the growth of Candida and to concentrate on eating a diet that maintains a healthy, balanced microbial ecosystem in the body. People try to rebalance their gut flora and relieve symptoms of Candida overgrowth by choosing foods wisely and avoiding those that contribute to it.

FUNDAMENTALS OF THE DIET FOR CANDIDA

The main idea behind the Candida diet is to stay away from foods that can encourage the growth of Candida yeast. These guidelines advise avoiding or consuming as little as possible processed food, high-carb foods, and sweets and sweeteners. These limitations are justified by the fact that Candida is a sugar bug and that eating a diet heavy in refined carbs can encourage the growth of Candida. By following these guidelines, people hope to establish an atmosphere that inhibits the growth of Candida and promotes a more balanced gut flora.

SWEETENERS AND SUGARS

One of the main tenets of the Candida diet is recognizing and steering clear of foods high in sugar and sweets. This covers both natural sweeteners like honey and maple syrup as well as refined sugars. The goal is to rob the Candida yeast of its main energy source because eating too much sugar is known to make Candida's overgrowth worse.

By eliminating these sugars, people hope to reduce the sustainability of the Candida population and promote the restoration of a more beneficial microbial balance in the gut.

PREPARED MEALS

Another food group that members of the Candida diet are recommended to stay away from is processed foods. Additives, preservatives, and other chemicals found in processed meals can upset the delicate balance of intestinal flora. Furthermore, a lot of processed meals have a lot of refined sugars and carbs, which create the perfect habitat for Candida to grow. On the Candida diet, people try to promote the restoration of a more varied and balanced microbiome by avoiding certain processed foods.

SUGAR-HIGH FOODS

On the Candida diet, foods high in carbohydrates—especially those with a high glycemic index—are not advised. These consist of white bread, refined grains, and some starchy veggies. Restricting high-carb foods makes sense because they can spike blood sugar levels quickly, which can foster Candida overgrowth. People who focus on complex carbohydrates, which are found in whole grains and vegetables, and choose lower-carb substitutes, hope to control their blood sugar levels and prevent the growth of Candida.

FOODS THAT FIGHT FUNGI

The Candida diet places more emphasis on including particular foods that can help prevent Candida overgrowth than it does on foods to avoid. Foods high in antifungal compounds, such as oregano, coconut oil, and garlic, may be able to stop Candida from growing. It is believed that incorporating these foods into the diet would help to naturally manage the overabundance of Candida and promote a better microbial balance in the gut.

RICH IN PROBIOTIC FOODS

Foods high in probiotics are also essential to the Candida diet. These foods supply the gut with good bacteria, such as yogurt, kefir, sauerkraut, and other fermented foods.

The intention is to increase the number of beneficial bacteria that can outcompete and inhibit the growth of Candida. People try to cultivate a more robust and diverse gut microbiota by including foods high in probiotics in their diet, which makes the environment less conducive to Candida overgrowth.

The Candida diet centers on deliberate food selections meant to minimize the elements that lead to Candida overgrowth while fostering the environment necessary for a well-balanced and robust gut flora.

People try to control symptoms and maintain general gut health by learning how diet affects Candida and following the guidelines of the diet.

CHAPTER FOUR

MAKING A MEAL PLAN SUITABLE FOR CANDIDA

ORGANIZING BALANCED MEALS

To promote general health and assist in controlling Candida overgrowth, developing a meal plan that is Candida-friendly requires careful consideration of the nutritional balance. Healthy fats, proteins, and carbs are examples of macronutrients that should be included in a well-rounded meal. Give special attention to whole, high-nutrient diets that supply vital vitamins and minerals. A balanced diet can be achieved by including lean proteins, complex carbohydrates, and a range of vibrant vegetables. Processed foods and refined sugars should be avoided since they may worsen Candida's symptoms.

EXAMPLE MEAL PLANS

An example of a Candida-friendly meal plan might be a vegetarian omelet with tomatoes and spinach for breakfast, grilled chicken salad with mixed greens for lunch, and baked salmon with steamed broccoli and quinoa for supper. Cucumber slices with hummus or celery sticks with nut butter could be snacks. The secret is to follow Candida-friendly guidelines and provide fun and diverse food. Keeping the diet varied through experimentation with food pairings might enhance general health.

BREAKFAST IDEAS

Think about including meals that are good in nutrients and low in sugar for breakfast. A smoothie consisting of berries, unsweetened almond milk, and a dollop of protein powder might be a filling choice. A pudding made with chia seeds, coconut milk, and cinnamon could be an additional option. These choices encourage a healthy start to the day by offering vital nutrients without feeding Candida.

LUNCH OPTIONS

A combination of healthy fats, non-starchy vegetables, and lean proteins can be had for lunch. Salads made of grilled chicken or tofu, mixed with bright vegetables, and dressed with a homemade dressing of lemon and olive oil can be a tasty and healthy option for those with Candida. A quinoa meal loaded with avocado and roasted veggies is a nutrient-dense substitute. It's critical to concentrate on components that support gut health and inhibit the growth of Candida.

DINNER RECIPES

There are many different options to choose from when creating a meal plan that is Candida-friendly. A tasty option is baked fish flavored with garlic and herbs and served with cauliflower rice and sautéed greens. A filling and healthy dinner option is a stir-fried turkey and vegetables with ginger and coconut aminos. Garlic, onions, and anti-fungal herbs can be used in dishes to enhance flavor and help prevent Candida overgrowth.

SNACK IDEAS

When it comes to snacks, a Candida-friendly diet calls for selecting foods that are high in nutrients and low in sugar. Nuts that are raw, like walnuts or almonds, can add a nice crunch and beneficial fats. Another delicious and healthy snack option is a small serving of Greek yogurt topped with a sprinkling of cinnamon, or you may try veggie sticks with guacamole. These choices support energy maintenance in between meals without sacrificing the overall meal plan's Candida-friendly guidelines.

CHAPTER FIVE

HERBS AND SUPPLEMENTS FOR THE TREATMENT OF CANDIDA

A SYNOPSIS OF SUPPLEMENTS

The treatment of candida frequently entails a multimodal strategy that includes dietary adjustments, lifestyle alterations, and the use of different vitamins and herbs. The goals of these complementary approaches are to promote general health and restore equilibrium to the body's microbial ecosystem. In this regard, vitamins are essential for treating Candida overgrowth and encouraging a more balanced internal environment.

ANTIBIOTICS

One important component of managing Candida is probiotics. These are good bacteria that support the equilibrium of the gut microbiota. By preventing the proliferation of dangerous bacteria like Candida, probiotics contribute to the maintenance of a balanced microbial ecology. For promoting gut health, strains like Lactobacillus and Bifidobacterium are very advantageous. Supplementing with probiotics can help restore the microbial equilibrium that has been upset by things like antibiotic use or a diet heavy in carbohydrates.

HERBS AND SUPPLEMENTS WITH ANTIFUNGALS

Antifungal herbs and vitamins are frequently used in conjunction with probiotics to control Candida. These natural substances have qualities that can aid in preventing Candida from growing and encouraging a more harmonious population of microorganisms. Herbs with antifungal properties include grapefruit seed extract, garlic, and oregano oil. These herbs are beneficial supplements to an all-encompassing Candida care strategy since they frequently include chemicals with antifungal, antibacterial, and antiviral qualities.

ADDITIONAL HELPFUL NUTRIENTS

In addition, other beneficial nutrients are essential for bolstering the body's defenses and creating an atmosphere that is less favorable for Candida overgrowth. It is well-recognized that some nutrients, like zinc, selenium, and vitamin C, strengthen the immune system. To stop Candida from growing and preserve a balanced population of microorganisms, a strong immune system is essential. When required, supplements can be taken in addition to a well-balanced diet to acquire these nutrients.

A healthy gut lining depends on the preservation of mucosal integrity, which is facilitated by particular nutrients in addition to immunological support. For instance, glutamine is an amino acid that is essential for maintaining the integrity of the intestinal lining and assisting in the prevention of pathogens, such as Candida, from entering the circulation.

Controlling Candida overgrowth necessitates a multifaceted strategy that extends beyond dietary modifications. Probiotics, antifungal herbs, and supportive minerals are just a few examples of supplements that are essential for balancing the gut flora, bolstering the immune system, and improving general health. It's crucial to remember that each person may react differently to supplements, so it's best to speak with a healthcare provider before adding any new ingredients to a plan for managing Candida.

CHAPTER SIX

LIFESTYLE TECHNIQUES TO MANAGE CANDIDA

STRESS REDUCTION

Reducing stress levels is essential to preventing Candida overgrowth. Prolonged stress can weaken the immune system, increasing the body's vulnerability to infections, such as Candida. The body's stress reaction can be controlled by incorporating stress-reduction methods including yoga, deep breathing exercises, and mindfulness meditation. A well-rested body is better able to handle daily pressures, which is another way that adequate sleep and stress management are closely related. People can establish a more resilient internal environment that is less conducive to Candida proliferation by addressing and controlling their stress.

SLEEPING HABITS

Getting enough sleep is essential for good health in general, and when it comes to controlling Candida, it is especially important to practice good sleep hygiene. Lack of sleep can impair immunity, increasing the body's vulnerability to diseases. Good sleep hygiene includes reducing screen time before bed, making a pleasant sleeping environment, and establishing a regular sleep pattern. Better immune function eventually supports the body's ability to control Candida. Addressing any underlying sleep issues or disturbances can also help.

CANDIDA AND EXERCISE

Frequent exercise helps reduce Candida in addition to being good for physical fitness. Exercise supports the body's detoxifying processes, strengthens the immune system, and improves circulation. When taken as a whole, these elements work to make the interior milieu less conducive to Candida's overgrowth. It's crucial to find a balance because too much or too severe exercise may cause the body to become stressed and weaken the immune system. Including strength training, flexibility training, and aerobic exercise in a regimen can be a comprehensive way to support general health and help prevent Candida-related problems.

HYDRATION AND CLEANSING

Maintaining adequate hydration is essential for assisting the body's detoxification processes, which can help with Candida control. Water facilitates the removal of compounds that could support an environment that is favorable to Candida overgrowth by flushing away toxins and waste products. Herbal teas and detoxifying drinks can be helpful in addition to water. Eating a diet high in antioxidant-rich foods, like fruits and vegetables, helps the body fight off free radicals and lessen oxidative stress. A diet rich in nutrients and well-rounded can support hydration efforts and create an environment within the body that inhibits the growth of Candida. Reducing alcohol, sugar, and processed food consumption can also help with detoxification and general health.

Lifestyle interventions aimed at controlling Candida involve an all-encompassing strategy that encompasses stress management, exercise, hydration, sleep hygiene, and detoxification.

CHAPTER SEVEN

OVERCOMING OBSTACLES AND FAILURES

HANDLING THE SYMPTOMS OF DETOX

Making healthy lifestyle adjustments is a frequent step on any road to overcoming obstacles and failures, and detoxification is one such step. The body may experience both physical and psychological detox symptoms while it gets used to a new routine. These symptoms, which might include everything from headaches and exhaustion to irritation, are frequently signs that the body is detoxifying. It is essential to recognize and accept the discomfort as a sign of growth rather than a setback to go through this phase successfully.

People might confront detox symptoms with a resilient mindset when they comprehend their nature. During this phase, staying hydrated is essential since drinking enough water helps the body's natural detoxifying processes. Incorporating foods high in nutrients can also supply vital vitamins and minerals that support the removal of pollutants. Having a network of friends, family, or online communities to lean on eases the transition through the symptoms of detoxification by providing a sense of support and common experiences.

GETTING AROUND IN SOCIAL SITUATIONS

Social settings can provide particular difficulties, particularly for those who are trying to bounce back after failures. To keep a positive outlook, it is essential to handle such situations with poise and assurance. To establish mutual understanding among peers and to articulate personal boundaries and goals, communication becomes an essential instrument. Having frank and open discussions about one's struggles can help one build a network of support that promotes personal development.

The secret to overcoming possible setbacks in social encounters is to have reasonable expectations. It's critical to understand that not every social event will support one's present goals, and it's acceptable to put one's own needs first. Learning coping mechanisms, such as practicing mindfulness or having a partner, who holds you accountable, can help people deal with social situations in a resilient way. People can overcome obstacles in social circumstances by being aware of and committed to their personal goals.

HANDLING DIE-OFF REACTIONS IN CANDIDA

Resolving underlying health issues is often necessary to overcome setbacks, and candida overgrowth is a prevalent issue that many people encounter. Die-off reactions might happen to people who are starting a journey to rid their bodies of excess candida. These reactions, which might include weariness, digestive problems, and flu-like symptoms, can be disheartening, but they are a sign that the overgrowth is being fought off.

A comprehensive strategy that includes dietary adjustments, specific supplements, and self-care routines is needed to manage candida die-off reactions. The key to slowing down the growth of the yeast is to follow an anti-candida diet that limits sugar and refined carbohydrate intake. Supplements with antifungal properties and probiotics can help the body fight candida overgrowth.

Furthermore, putting enough sleep and stress management first promotes general well-being and lessens the severity of die-off reactions.

Overcoming obstacles and failures requires a multimodal strategy that handles social situations, treats detox symptoms, and manages candida die-off reactions.

CHAPTER EIGHT

PROLONGED UPKEEP AND INTERVENTION

Maintaining and preventing health problems over the long term frequently entails a multimodal approach that includes introducing foods gradually, closely observing and evaluating the patient's progress, and putting preventative measures in place to stop the recurrence of particular conditions, like Candida overgrowth.

REINTRODUCING FOODS GRADUALLY

Reintroducing foods gradually is essential for long-term maintenance, especially for those who have experienced dietary interventions or limitations. When reintroducing foods gradually, the body can adjust and the likelihood of negative reactions is reduced, whether the goal is controlling allergies, intolerances, or adhering to a particular therapeutic diet. This procedure is necessary to maintain a varied and balanced diet as well as to find potential triggers that may have previously contributed to health problems.

TRACKING AND EVALUATING DEVELOPMENT

A vital part of preserving long-term health is tracking and evaluating improvement. Tracking changes in health status is made easier with the use of self-assessment tools, health screenings, and routine checkups. By taking a proactive stance, people and healthcare providers can spot new problems early on, deal with them quickly, and modify their plans as necessary. Monitoring can include keeping track of vital signs, test findings, and subjective markers of well-being to guarantee a thorough assessment of general health.

KEEPING CANDIDA FROM RECURRING

Targeted therapies and continuous observation are needed to stop the recurrence of Candida overgrowth. Yeasts like Candida can cause infections when they proliferate too much inside the body, which can result in several health problems. People may need to stick to their antifungal medication regimen, eat a low-sugar diet, and lead a healthy, immune-supporting lifestyle to prevent recurrence. Identifying the risk factors and triggers of Candida overgrowth is essential to creating a customized preventative strategy.

A holistic approach to health is essential for long-term maintenance and prevention, in addition to targeted therapies. This entails taking care of lifestyle elements including stress reduction, consistent exercise, and enough sleep. These components support general health and have a beneficial impact on the body's capacity to keep equilibrium and fend off a variety of health issues.

The long-term maintenance and prevention of health problems involve a variety of tactics, such as the careful reintroduction of foods, close observation of development, and focused actions to stop the recurrence of particular ailments like Candida overgrowth.

Through the integration of these methods with a comprehensive perspective on health, people can develop long-lasting routines that enhance their overall wellness.

CHAPTER NINE

RECIPES FOR THE DIET OF CANDIDA

RECIPES FOR BREAKFAST

Carefully choosing components is necessary to make filling and healthy breakfast options that follow the Candida Diet. Think about including lean proteins, such as turkey or eggs, which offer a steady energy supply without encouraging Candida overgrowth. Almond flour pancakes or coconut flour muffins can make delicious grain-free substitutes. These recipes provide a delightful and satisfying way to start the day while also adhering to the diet's constraints.

Incorporating foods high in probiotics, such as unsweetened yogurt, can also help to preserve a balanced gut flora, which is essential for controlling Candida infection.

RECIPES FOR LUNCH AND DINNER

Developing lunch and dinner recipes that adhere to the Candida Diet requires making calculated decisions that give low-sugar and anti-inflammatory components priority. A satisfying supper can consist of grilled chicken or fish and a range of non-starchy vegetables. Playing around with herbs and spices improves the dish's flavor and strengthens its anti-Candida qualities. Traditional grains can be easily swapped out for zucchini noodles or cauliflower rice, which keeps the dish Candida-friendly. Adding nutritious fats, like avocado or olive oil, to meals enhances their nutritional value and creates a satisfying mealtime experience.

DESSERTS AND SNACKS

When following the Candida Diet, finding creative ways to satiate desires without going overboard with diet limitations is necessary when choosing snacks and desserts. Nuts that are raw, like walnuts and almonds, can make a filling and easy snack because they are high in protein and healthy fats. Raw vegetable sticks with homemade hummus or guacamole make a cool, Candida-friendly substitute for packaged munchies. For desserts, looking into recipes that use almond or coconut flour as a base can produce delicious delights that follow the rules of the Candida Diet. You may add sweetness guilt-free by using natural sweeteners like stevia or monk fruit, which won't promote Candida overgrowth.